Health Technical Memorandum 2040

Good practice guide

The control of legionellae in healthcare premises – a code of practice

London: HMSO

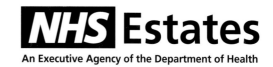

NHS Estates

An Executive Agency of the Department of Health

Cover photograph:
Scanning electron micrograph of a biofilm on latex showing
amoeba grazing the bacterial consortium (magnification x 1440).
Reproduced by kind permission of Julie Rogers and A B Dowsett,
Public Health Laboratory Service Centre for Applied Microbiology
and Research, Porton Down, Salisbury, Wiltshire.

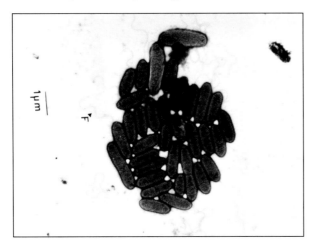

Above:
A colony of bacteria *Legionella pneumophila*. The bacteria are
non-sporing, typically 2–3 μm long, 0.3–0.9 μm wide. Flagella,
which can be clearly seen, provide mobility of the organism.
Reproduced by kind permission of Public Health Laboratory
Service Centre for Applied Microbiology and Research.

HMSO
Standing order service

Placing a standing order with HMSO BOOKS enables a
customer to receive future titles in this series automatically
as published. This saves the time, trouble and expense of
placing individual orders and avoids the problem of
knowing when to do so. For details please write to HMSO
BOOKS (PC 13A/1), Publications Centre, PO Box 276,
London SW8 5DT quoting reference 14 02 017.
The standing order service also enables customers to receive
automatically as published all material of their choice which
additionally saves extensive catalogue research. The scope
and selectivity of the service has been extended by new
techniques, and there are more than 3,500 classifications to
choose from. A special leaflet describing the service in detail
may be obtained on request.

About this publication

Health Technical Memorandum (HTM) 2040 provides recommendations, advice and guidance on controlling legionellae in healthcare premises. It is applicable to new and existing sites, and is for use at various stages during the inception, design, upgrading, refurbishment, extension and maintenance of a building.

HTM 2040 focuses on the:

   a. legal and mandatory requirements;

   b. design of systems;

   c. maintenance of systems;

   d. operation of systems.

It is published as five separate volumes, each addressing a specialist discipline:

   a. **Management policy** – outlines the overall responsibility of managers of healthcare premises, and details their legal and mandatory obligations. It summarises the essential background information required to understand the principles of the control of legionellae. This is followed by an epidemiology of legionellosis, essential to understanding the rationale behind the various control and design measures advocated in succeeding volumes. A management checklist is provided in the Appendix to this volume; it lists the major tasks and should form the basis of a risk assessment;

   b. **Design considerations** – highlights the overall requirements and considerations that should be applied to the design up to the contract document;

   c. **Validation and verification** – considers the testing and commissioning aspects, also providing guidance on the identification of problem areas;

   d. **Operational management** – considers aspects of preventing and controlling legionellae. It also contains information on the operation, maintenance and cleaning of evaporative cooling towers;

e. this volume – **Good practice guide** – gives advice on the course of action if an outbreak of legionnaires' disease is suspected, on cleaning and disinfection of a cooling tower implicated in an outbreak of legionnaires' disease, and on the use of sodium hypochlorite solutions for chlorination of cooling water systems in hospitals. Further advice is given in the form of:

(i) emptying times for cooling tower ponds;

(ii) a questionnaire to assess the serviceability of existing cooling systems;

(iii) a sample logbook for the planned maintenance of a cooling tower.

Guidance in this Health Technical Memorandum is complemented by the library of National Health Service Model Engineering Specifications. Users of the guidance are advised to refer to the relevant specifications.

The contents of this HTM in terms of management policy, operational policy and technical guidance are endorsed by:

a. the Welsh Office for the NHS in Wales;

b. the Health and Personal Social Services Management Executive in Northern Ireland;

c. the National Health Service in Scotland Management Executive;

and they set standards consistent with Departmental Cost Allowances.

This HTM was written with the advice and assistance of experts in the NHS and industry.

References to legislation appearing in the main text of this guidance apply in England and Wales. Where references differ for Scotland and/or Northern Ireland these are given in marginal notes.

Where appropriate, marginal notes are also used to amplify the text.

Contents

Appendix 1 – The use of sodium hypochlorite solutions for chlorination of cooling water systems in hospitals

1.1 Chlorine is an excellent and fast-acting biocide, widely used for controlling microbial growth in cooling waters of wet, evaporative heat exchangers. However, it is essential to note the following four facts, which determine its efficiency during use:

a. chlorine has no detergent cleansing powers. It is essential that slime and debris are removed by thorough cleansing before chlorine is used, otherwise micro-organisms will survive disinfection as a result of the physical shielding afforded by these slimes;

b. chlorine is a highly reactive chemical and will very rapidly combine with organic matter, ammonium compounds and any oxidisable materials (for example ferrous and manganous salts, hydrogen sulphide) present in the water or on wetted surfaces. These reactions will greatly reduce, or even neutralise completely, the disinfecting power. In practice, the level of free available residual chlorine (that is, that available for disinfection) will always be less than that calculated from the dose added, and will decline progressively after addition. For these reasons, chlorine should only be used in systems which are already clean, and the level of free available residual chlorine in the water must always be checked after adding chlorine and allowing it to become completely mixed with the circulating water;

c. chlorine should not be used with other biocides, since they may neutralise each other, unless they are known to be compatible;

d. the disinfecting effect is greater at pH values at or below the neutral pH value of 7.0. Temperature will also affect the efficacy. At pH values above 8.0, the disinfecting power is greatly reduced. This is because the disinfecting activity is mainly brought about by hypochlorous acid ($HOCl$), which exists in pH-dependent equilibrium with hypochlorite ions ($OCl-$), in solution. For example, in water at 30°C and pH 7, 71% free available residual chlorine will exist as hypochlorous acid, whereas at pH 9 there will be only 2.4% hypochlorous acid, and 97.6% will be in the form of hypochlorite ion $OCl-$, which is not as powerful a disinfectant as $HOCl$ (see Figure 1, Effect of pH on chlorination (as $HOCl$)).

Sodium hypochlorite and available chlorine

1.2 Sodium hypochlorite solutions are the most suitable for chlorinating hospital and other cooling waters. Other chemicals such as bleaching powder ("chloride of lime"), "high-test hypochlorite" or "slow-release tablets" (chloro-isocyanurate compounds) are less convenient to prepare or use, and liquefied chlorine gas is too hazardous.

1.3 Sodium hypochlorite solutions are sold containing 10–15 per cent available chlorine. They contain sodium hydroxide which helps to prevent degradation of the sodium hypochlorite during storage. The commercial preparation has a pH value of about 11 and also contains sodium chloride.

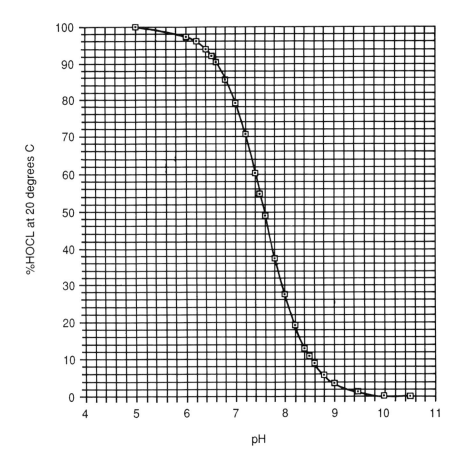

Figure 1   Effect of pH on chlorination (as HOCl)

1.4   It is conventional to express the strengths of chlorine compounds and similar oxidising disinfectants in terms of "available chlorine". This is for analytical convenience, since it provides a common reference of oxidising power for various chemicals used in disinfection of water (for example chlorine, hypochlorous acid, hypochlorite ion, chloramines, chlorine dioxide and sulphur dioxide). Chlorine itself (Cl_2) is assumed to be 100 per cent available.

1.5   Commercial sodium hypochlorite solution contains 10–15 per cent (w/v) available chlorine, representing a dilution of about 10 to 7 times respectively.

1.6   In tests of treated water for the presence of free available residual chlorine, the hypochlorous acid and hypochlorite ion both react by oxidation, so both are measured. This makes it easy to determine the dose of available chlorine added by calculating the dilution (as shown in Table 1).

1.7   This table does not allow for deterioration in strength of the hypochlorite solution, or for chlorine demand within the water and the cooling circuit. Hence, the actual concentration of free available residual chlorine in the water must always be checked after the dose has been added and properly mixed with the cooling water.

Care in storage and use of sodium hypochlorite solutions

1.8 Solutions must be stored in a dark, cool, well-ventilated place and handled with care according to instructions on the label. They must not be stored or mixed with other chemicals such as acids, ammonia, ammoniacal compounds or cleaning materials because of the risks of evolution of poisonous, chlorine gas and the spontaneous formation of explosive nitrogen trichloride. The solutions are caustic, causing burns to the eyes and skin, are poisonous and will rapidly bleach and rot clothing and woodwork and corrode metals. They must only be placed in glass or plastic containers. When handled, waterproof protective clothing and eyeshields must be worn. Any splashes on the eyes, skin or clothing should be washed off immediately with plenty of cold water. If swallowed, medical advice should be sought immediately. Further information on the safe handling of sodium hypochlorite solutions is given in the Department of the Environment's publication, 'Swimming Pool Disinfection Systems Using Sodium Hypochlorite – Guidelines for Design and Operation' (DOE, 1979).

Chlorination of hospital cooling water systems to suppress bacterial growth

Routine chlorination as an alternative to other biocides

1.9 If chlorine (or biocides) is/are not added to the cooling-water circuits, legionellae and other micro-organisms may become established because of the favourable operating temperature range and if sufficient nutrients are present. Nutrients may be derived from such sources as contaminated make-up water, dust, leaves, bird droppings and from decaying microbial slime. Low concentrations of free available residual chlorine will prevent growth of legionellae and other micro-organisms, thereby preventing the build-up of slimes even if nutrients are present in the water. The concentration of free available residual chlorine needed to suppress microbial growth will depend upon the quality of the water being circulated and the condition of pipework.

1.10 It is essential that the chosen level is maintained since the free chlorine will be absorbed constantly by organic matter and microbial growth in the system – and lost by chemical degradation when the water cascades through the tower packing. Experience has shown that control is achieved when the free available residual chlorine level is maintained constantly at 1–2 mg/l, and to avoid corrosion, a level of 3 mg/l is the maximum which should be permitted.

1.11 Where continuous dosing and control is not possible, it may be possible to maintain a similar level of control by dosing intermittently (not less frequently than weekly), to achieve an initial level of 10 mg/l as free available residual chlorine, after allowing for the solution to become completely mixed with the cooling water. If the level falls below 1 mg/l before the next dosing, the frequency of dosing should be increased.

Periodic cleaning and disinfection of the cooling circuit

1.12 Because sodium hypochlorite in solution has no detergent or penetrative properties, the aim must be to use thorough mechanical cleaning with brushing and rinsing to remove slime and debris before the system is disinfected and returned to service. The procedure outlined in this HTM is based upon practical engineering and microbiological experience such as described by Colbourne et al (1978).

1.13 The procedure recognises that disinfection is a function of both time and concentration. Practical experience in the water supply industry for disinfection of pipelines and storage reservoirs, within buildings and in ships, has shown that satisfactory disinfection of cleaned structures can be obtained if the concentration x time product (CT) is at least 50 mg h/l. To achieve this degree of treatment, the dose of available chlorine added, as calculated from Table 1, must be considerably in excess, to allow for chlorine demand. Table 2 indicates the actual dose of chlorine available which may have to be added to achieve a CT product of 50 mg h/l. Experience has shown that when doses of 20 mg/l or less are used, there is a risk of disinfection failure because of the effect of chlorine demand.

1.14 Provided that the procedure has been followed correctly, there is no benefit in extending the contact period. Indeed, if the procedure has been applied incorrectly and the level of chlorine is less than that required, increasing the contact time would create conditions where untreated water stagnated in a water system, thereby allowing time for bacterial regrowth. There is a risk of accelerating corrosion/deterioration of the materials of construction if chlorinated water is left to stand in pipework overnight on a repeated basis.

Required dose of available chlorine (mg/l)	Volume of sodium hypochlorite to be added		
	ml/m^3	fluid oz 1000 gal	ml/1000 gal
1	10	1.6	45
5	50	8	227
10	100	16	454
50	500	80	2270

Table 1 Approximate amounts of commercial sodium hypochlorite solution (10% (w/v) available chlorine) to be added to achieve a given dose

Dose to be added		Typical measured free available residual chlorine (mg/l)		
As chlorine mg/l	As hypochlorite 10% w/v available chlorine (ml/m^3)	Contact period (h)	immediately after addition	after contact period
50	500	1	40–50	30
40	400	1.5	30–40	25
30	300	2	20–30	15
20	200	3.5	10–15	5
15	150	5	5–10	5

Table 2 Examples of the dose of available chlorine which may be needed initially to achieve disinfection to a concentration x time product of 50 mg h/l

Appendix 2 – Questionnaire: Assessment of serviceability of existing cooling systems

Northern Ireland: Equivalent provisions are proposed for Northern Ireland

1. Are they registered with local authority?

2. Siting of cooling tower

a. Is the cooling tower located near a fresh-air intake to an air conditioning or ventilation system?

b. Is it possible for wind to carry the cooling tower discharge vapour towards the windows of a nearby area or department where there are patients?

c. Is the siting such that good access is available for maintenance purposes?

d. Is the siting or tower configuration such that wind could cause reversal of air flow and spray to carry over from the air-inlet louvres?

3. Cooling tower

a. Are all the internal parts of the cooling tower readily accessible, or can they be rendered so?

b. Is corrosion apparent either internally or externally?

c. Is fouling apparent within the tower?

d. Is debris, sludge or slime apparent in the tower water?

e. Are the drift eliminators closely fitting and firmly seated in their support grid?

f. Is the pack, or any other part of the tower, manufactured from natural materials such as timber?

g. Are natural rubbers used as seals or gaskets in the spray system or elsewhere?

h. When operating at full load, is excessive drift visible from the tower discharge?

j. Is there a coarse strainer located over the outflow pipe from the tower?

k. Is the drain from the pond piped to discharge above a gulley connected to the foul water drain system?

m. Is the overflow from the pond piped to discharge above a gulley connected to the foul water drainage system?

n. Is there a readily accessible pond water sampling point available?

p. Is there a readily accessible water sampling point available to sample tower make-up water?

q. Is there a strict water treatment programme in operation to control:

    (i) TDS;

    (ii) pH;

(iii)   total hardness;

(iv)   chlorides;

(v)   scale;

(vi)   slime;

(vii)   water treatment chemical/additive levels;

(viii)   corrosion;

(ix)   sludge;

(x)   algae;

(xi)   micro-organisms?

r.   Is the tower and the entire distribution system cleaned and disinfected at the correct intervals?

s.   Is there a regular maintenance programme and recording/logbook system in operation?

t.   Is a water meter installed on the feed to the make-up valve? Is it accurate?

4.   The distribution system

a.   Is the pipework distribution system clearly visible and accessible?

b.   Is the pipework system easily dismantled for inspection or is it provided with inspection points?

c.   Is there a risk of water stagnation in the pipeline strainer assembly? (This can occur with duplicate sets if precautions against stagnation are not taken.)

d.   Is there a risk of water stagnation in the maintenance bypass across the 3-way control valve? (This will occur if the bypass valve is fully closed. Flow should be encouraged or the bypass removed.)

e.   Where duplicate pumps are installed, do they alternate on a daily basis?

f.   Are there adequate manual drain points installed, with drain discharge lines piped to discharge above a gully connected to the foul water drainage system?

g.   Are there adequate, readily accessible water sampling points installed in the distribution system?

h.   Is the automatic TDS drain line piped to discharge above a gulley connected to the foul water drainage system?

j.   Are there adequate thermometers and pressure gauges installed to enable system performance to be monitored and understood?

k.   Is a regular maintenance programme and recording/logbook system in operation?

l.   Does an internal inspection of the condenser and pipework system indicate fouling is present?

Appendix 3 – The course of action if an outbreak of legionnaires' disease is suspected

The hospital outbreak control team (the team) should include the consultant in communicable disease control

3.1 The nominated person will usually be informed of a suspected case of legionnaires' disease possibly associated with healthcare premises by either the outbreak control team or the local Consultant in Communicable Disease Control (CCDC). If a case is suspected, then the hospital outbreak team will normally work in association with the Public Health Laboratory Service and the local CCDC to search for the source of the causative organism. It is essential that systems are not drained or disinfected before samples have been taken. The nominated person's role is an important one – guiding the team to the various water systems within the building and, in particular, to the points from which samples can be taken. Easy access to these sampling points is essential.

3.2 The investigation will concentrate upon all potential sources of legionella infection, including:

- the domestic hot and cold water distribution system;
- wet spray cooling water systems;
- showers or spray washing equipment;
- drainage systems and traps;
- spas, whirlpool baths or therapy pools;
- humidifiers in ventilation systems;
- cooling coils in air-conditioning systems;
- fountains and sprinklers.

3.3 To assist in such investigations, the nominated person must be able to provide details of all associated equipment, including all documentation. He/she must assist by advising the investigating team on the extent of servicing on the site, and by locating taps and sample points.

3.4 The nominated person must also identify the locations of any medical equipment used for dental care, respiratory therapy and within haemodialysis units, etc.

3.5 Off-site information will also be required, such as whether there have been any local excavation or earthmoving works, alterations to water supply systems, or drainage systems or any other factors which may have a bearing on the site.

3.6 The address and telephone number of the nearest weather station will be required – this is likely to be a local airport, university or college department.

3.7 The team is responsible for identifying the cause of infection, and will advise on cleaning, disinfection, any modifications, and long-term control measures.

Appendix 4 – Sample logbook

Logbook No ......

Establishment   ....

                                                 ....

Site   ....

                                                 ....

                                                 ....

                                                 ....

Installation   Evaporative cooling water system

                                                 Located ....

                                                 Serving ....

Appendix 4 – Sample logbook

Establishment .... Logbook

Site .... Page No 1

Installation .... Serial No 1

Frequency..........

Typical evaporative cooling tower system arrangement

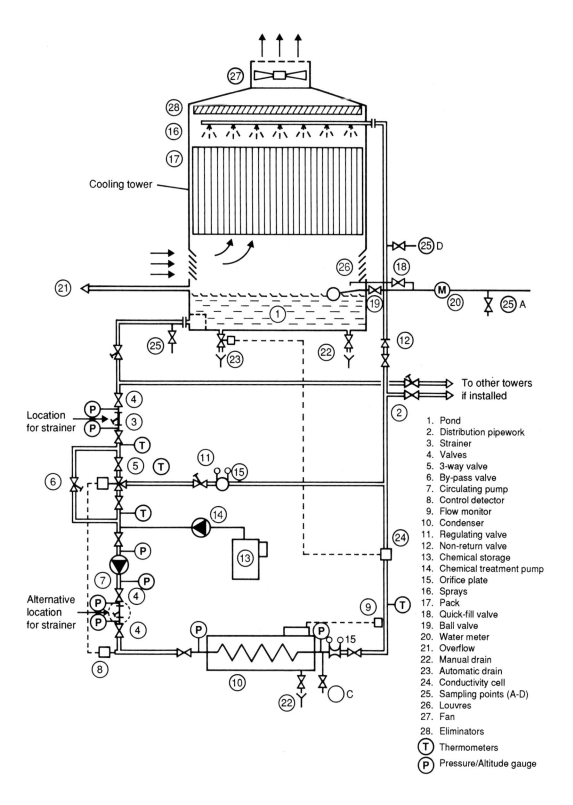

Cooling tower

1. Pond
2. Distribution pipework
3. Strainer
4. Valves
5. 3-way valve
6. By-pass valve
7. Circulating pump
8. Control detector
9. Flow monitor
10. Condenser
11. Regulating valve
12. Non-return valve
13. Chemical storage
14. Chemical treatment pump
15. Orifice plate
16. Sprays
17. Pack
18. Quick-fill valve
19. Ball valve
20. Water meter
21. Overflow
22. Manual drain
23. Automatic drain
24. Conductivity cell
25. Sampling points (A-D)
26. Louvres
27. Fan
28. Eliminators

(T) Thermometers

(P) Pressure/Altitude gauge

Location for strainer

Alternative location for strainer

To other towers if installed

Establishment . . . . Logbook

Site . . . . Page No 1

Installation . . . . Serial No 2

Frequency. . . . .

Operation

Water is circulated to the condenser at a constant temperature of 25°C. This temperature is achieved by modulation of the 3 way control valve (item 5) missing proportions of water from the cooling tower or bypass line as controlled by the detector (Item 8).

Schedule of commissioning data

Cooling tower rating . . . . kW
Air on   28°C db   21°C wb   Air off . . . °C db . . . . . . °Cwb
Air volume . . . . m3/   Pressure difference . . . . Pa
Water temperature on . . . . °C,
off . . . . °C
Water flow rate . . . . l/s

Circulating pump

Flow rate . . . . l/s   Suction pressure . . . . bar
Static pressure . . . . bar   Discharge pressure . . . . bar

Refrigeration condenser

Rating . . . . kW
Water on . . . . °C
off . . . . °C
Pressure drop . . . . kPa

System volume

Pipework distribution . . . . litres
Cooling tower . . . . litres
Total volume . . . . litres

Plant operating times

Hours per day . . . . hrs
on . . . . hrs
off . . . . hrs
Days per week . . . . days
Weeks per year . . . . weeks
State normal operating season _____ from _____ to _____

System circulation time

$$\frac{\text{Total volume in litres}}{\text{Pump flow rate l/s} \times 60} = \quad .. \text{ mins*}$$

*   Due to short-circuiting within the pond, a complete change of pond water cannot be guaranteed within this theoretical period, which should be used as a guide only.

Total dissolved solid (TDS) control

Desired control level . . . .$\mu s/m^2$
Method of control   for example conductivity control

Chemical treatment system A

Chemical formulation . . . .
Holding tank volume . . . . litres
Pump duty . . . . l/hr @ . . . . kPa
Method of control . . . .

Chemical treatment system B

Chemical formulation . . . .
Holding tank volume . . . . litres
Pump duty . . . . l/hr @ . . . . kPa
Method of control . . . .

Chemical treatment system C

Chemical formulation . . . .
Holding tank volume . . . . litres
Pump duty . . . . l/hr @ . . . . kPa
Method of control . . . .

Chemical treatment system D

Chemical formulation . . . .
Holding tank volume . . . . litres
Pump duty . . . . l/hr @ . . . . kPa
Method of control . . . .

Chemical treatment system E

Chemical formulation . . . .
Holding tank volume . . . . litres
Pump duty . . . . l/hr @ . . . . kPa
Method of control . . . .

Establishment .... Logbook

Site .... Page No 2

Installation .... Serial No 1

Frequency W & M

Evaporative cooling system operational checks

(W = weekly, M = monthly)

Note as applicable: S = satisfactory ;   N/S = not satisfactory.
Record defects over page.

Item	Design Data	Fre-quency	Date of inspection							
1. Refrigeration M/C:										
a) water in/out °C		W								
b) temp. diff. °C		W								
c) current drawn A		W								
d) pressure drop kPa		W								
e) observations										
2. Condenser water pump										
a) outlet press bar		W								
b) suction press bar		W								
c) diff. pressure bar		W								
d) duty/standby		W								
e) hours run Pump 1		W								
f) hours run Pump 2		W								
g) full load current A		W								
h) observations										
3. Control valve (range 0-10)										
a) valve position (0-10)		W								
b) temp. from tower °C		W								
c) temp. at detector °C		W								
d) manual operation		W								
e) observations										
Inspector's signature										

Item	Design data	Fre-quency	Date of inspection								
4. Tower											
a) pond inspection											
b) ball valve operation		W									
c) fan/speed r.p.m.		W									
d) fan current		W									
e) air on °C wb		W									
f) fan operation check		W									
g) casing check		W									
h) moisture carry over		W									
j) overflow check		W									
k) strainer check		W									
m) pond heater current		W									
operational check		W									
n) sump current drawn											
p) drift eliminator		W									
check		M									
q) pack check											
r) discharge ducting		M									
check (if applicable)		M									
s) NR damper check											
(if applicable)		M									
t) spray/spare/trough											
check		M									
u) inlet louvre check											
v) observations		M									
5. Circulation system											
a) strainer pressure											
drop kPa		M									
b) drains											
c) valves		W									
d) vents		W									
e) pipework		W									
f) leaks		W									
g) flow to tower (with 3		W									
way valve fully open)		M									
h) flow to system											
(with 3 way valve in		M									
full recirc.)											
j) flow monitor check											
k) observations		W									
Inspector's signature											

Defects schedule				
Date	**Observation**	**Noted**	**Diagnosed cause of defect**	**Initials**

Defects schedule				
Date	Observations	Noted	Diagnosed cause of defect	Initials

Establishment . . . . Logbook

Site . . . . Page No 3

Installation . . . . Serial No 1

Frequency . . . .

**Operational tests on make-up water from
evaporative cooling systems**

Note as applicable: S = satisfactory;   N/S = not satisfactory.

Name of water undertaking . . . . Tel No . . . .
Name of water treatment contractor . . . . Tel No . . . .

Control parameters

Typical water usage . . . . litres
Normal tolerances ± . . . . litres
Total hardness . . . .   pH . . . .
Conductivity . . . .   Chlorides . . . .

Where installed, name of water softener device . . . .

Date	Water meter reading	Water used litres	Total hard-ness	Conduc-tivity	pH	TDS	Obser-vations	Initials

Defects schedule				
Date	**Observations**	**Noted**	**Diagnosed cause of defect**	**Initials**

Establishment . . . . Logbook

Site . . . . Page No 4

Installation . . . . Serial No 1

Frequency . . . .

**Detail sheet for water treatment programme
associated with evaporative cooling**

Name of water treatment   contractor . . . . **Date** . . . .
Cooling tower duty kW
Design operating conditions . . . . l/s
On . . . . **°C Off** . . . . °C
Plant operating period . . . . hrs/day
days/week . . . .
weeks/year . . . .
Total system water capacity . . . . litres
Evaporate rate . . . . l/s   **Peak daily output** . . . . . . litres
Pre-treatment plant . . . .
Bleed system control method . . **(for example conductivity control)**

Control parameters:

> **Conductivity** . . . .
> **TDS** . . . . typical
> **Chlorine** . . . . typical
> **pH** . . . . typical
> **Chlorides** . . . .

Selected chemical treatment				
Chemical formulation	**Initial dose**	**Maintenance dose**	**Dosing equipment**	
			Dilution rate	**Flow rate**
A				
B				
C				
D				
E				
F				

Chemical treatment criteria for proprietary products listed in table below

Treatment	Control units		* Units	Type of test	Remarks
(state A,B,C,D,E,F)	Min	Max			
System water					
Scale controller					
Corrosion inhib.					
Sludge dispensive					
pH					
Methyl orange alkalinity M					
TDS					
Biocide					

* Criteria concentrations are shown in mg/1 (p.p.m) in terms of $CaCO_3$ unless otherwise stated.

Table 3 Biological activity

Bacterial analytical procedure	General bacterial count max organisms per ml	Remarks

Establishment . . . . **Logbook**

Site . . . . **Page No 5**

Installation . . . . **Serial No 1**

. . . . Frequency . . . .

Operational tests on system water quality for
evaporative cooling system

Name of water treatment contractor . . . .
Note as applicable: S = satisfactory;   N/S = not satisfactory.
State defect over page.

Date	System water test ppm				System condition S or N/S	Chemicals dosed A,B,C,D,E, or F, state chemical and litres	Dosing equipment operation S or N/S	Initials
	Scale controls	Corrosion inhibitor	Sludge dispensive	Total ALK or pH				

Dosing system operational checks   Frequency - weekly

Item	Date of inspection							
1. Chemical treatment system A a) contents of holding tank (litres) b) volume of chemical used (litres/day) c) top up holding tank and record new volume (litres) d) pump operational check e) control device check f) pump duty check g) observations S or N/S								
2. Chemical treatment system B a) contents of holding tank (litres) b) volume of chemical used (litres/day) c) top up holding tank and record new volume (litres) d) pump operational check e) control device check f) pump duty check g) observations S or N/S								
3. Chemical treatment system C a) content of holding tank (litres) b) volume of chemical used (litres/day c) top up holding tank and record new volume (litres) d) pump operational check e) control device check f) pump duty check g) observations S or N/S								
Inspector's signature								

Defects schedule				
Date	Observation	Noted	Diagnosed cause of defect	Initials

Defects schedule				
Date	Observation	Noted	Diagnosed cause of defect	Initials

Establishment . . . . Logbook

Site . . . . Page No 6

Installation . . . . Serial No 1

Frequency   weekly

Maintenance sheet for cooling tower fans

When maintenance task is satisfactorily completed the operative is to tick the box opposite. If task cannot be completed due to mechanical failure, insert a cross in the box opposite and note defect on the observation sheet.

Job Description	Date of inspection							
1. Cooling tower No..... a) isolate electrical supply to fan. b) isolate condenser water pumps and/or valve to tower being serviced. c) remove fan guard and wipe clean motor, drive shaft and general parts to be serviced. d) adjust thrust and collar bearings e) lubricate fan bearing with .... shots of grease type .... f) lubricate motor bearing with .... shots of grease type .... g) check oil level in drive gearbox and top up as necessary using oil type .... h) lightly grease shafts and parts exposed to vapour as appropriate. i) if belted drive, check belt tension and adjust as necessary. j) reassemble guard and bring plant back into service. k) check ball valve assembly for correct operating level and adjust as necessary.								
Engineer's signature								

27

Defects schedule				
Date	Observations	Noted	Diagnosed cause of defect	Initials

Establishment . . . . Logbook

Site . . . . Page No 7

Installation . . . . Serial No 1

Frequency 3 monthly

Maintenance sheet for cooling tower
3 monthly tasks

When maintenance task is satisfactorily completed the operative is to tick the box opposite. If task cannot be completed due to mechanical failure, insert a cross in the box opposite and note defect on the observation sheet.

Job description	Date of inspection							
1. Cooling tower No..... a) isolate electrical supply to tower. b) isolate condenser water pumps and/or valve to tower being serviced. c) remove fan guard, wipe clean, inspect for rust spots, rub down apply rust inhibitor and paint. When replacing guard lightly grease holding bolts. d) clean fan casing, impeller, housing, holding bolts and framework. Inspect all steelwork for rust spots, rub down, apply rust inhibitor and paint. Apply protective grease to bolts and parts exposed to vapour. e) remove dirt eliminators, brush and wipe clean, apply hose as necessary. Inspect for signs of fouling. If fouling is present apply chemical dispersant and remove. Similarly clean eliminator support grid and housing. Inspect for signs of rust, rub down, apply rust inhibitor and paint. When complete replace eliminators taking care to place the correct way up, to align and seal to prevent moisture by -passing.								
Engineer's signature								

Job description	Date of inspection							
f) remove all spray nozzles and clean. Replace all suspect grommets and washers. If trough distribution system, remove trough and wipe clean, hose as necessary and rod through all nozzles. Inspect distribution pipe for signs of rust, rub down, apply rust inhibitor and paint.								
g) remove pack from tower and clean by scraping, wiping, brushing and application of hose. (Method to be sympathetic to material). If fouling is present use chemical dispersant to remove fouling or if more appropriate dispose of media and replace with new. Similarly clean inside of tower casing and pack support grid. Inspection for signs of rust, rub down, apply inhibitor and paint. When complete take care with replacement to ensure by-passing does not occur.								
h) clean louvres and screens. Inspect for signs of rust, rub down, apply inhibitor and paint.								
i) isolate ball valve and pond outflow pipe. Drain pond. Clean out debris and sediment, hose out pond until clear. Remove strainer and scrub clean. Clean outflow pipe orifice. Hose through all drain lines and sampling pipes. If fouling is present use chemical dispersant and remove. When clean and dry inspect pond for signs of rust, rub down, apply inhibitor and paint.								
Engineer's signature								

Defects schedule				
Date	**Observations**	**Noted**	**Diagnosed cause of defect**	**Initials**

Defects schedule				
Date	Observations	Noted	Diagnosed cause of defect	Initials

Establishment . . . . Logbook

Site . . . . Page No 7

Installation   Serial No 2

                                                                                              Frequency 3 monthly

Maintenance sheet for cooling tower
3 monthly tasks

When maintenance task is satisfactorily completed the operative is to tick the box opposite. If task cannot be completed due to mechanical failure, insert a cross in the box opposite and note defect on the observation sheet.

Job Description	Date of inspection							
j) clean ball valve assembly and adjust operating level as necessary. k) inspect immersion heater for signs of leaks and repair as necessary. Clean immersion heater coil and use chemical dispersant to remove any fouling. Inspect weatherproofing on all trace heating and insulation, and repair where damaged. Check tightness of all cable terminations.								
Engineer's signature								

Defects schedule				
Date	Observations	Noted	Diagnosed cause of defect	Initials

Establishment . . . . Logbook

Site . . . . Page No 7

Installation . . . . Serial No 3

Maintenance sheet for cooling towers
3 monthly tasks

**Frequency 3 months
and as necessary**

When maintenance task is satisfactorily completed the operative is to tick the box opposite. If task cannot be completed due to mechanical failure, insert a cross in the box opposite and note defect on the observation sheet.

Job Description	Date of inspection							
1. Fan assembly a) drain oil from gear box and replace using oil type......................								
2. Ball valve a) replace ball valve washer and readjust as necessary each alternate 3 months.								
3. Seasonal cleaning & disinfection a) carry out disinfection of make-up tank and distribution pipework as required by Code of Practice. Record quantity and sodium hypochlorite used for disinfection (litres). Record residual chlorine level after 1 hour standing duration (p.p.m.) b) carry out disinfection of tower and distribution system as required by Code of Practice. Record quantity of sodium hypochlorite used for disinfection (litres). Record residual chlorine level after 4 hour circulation period (p.p.m.) c) bring system back into service.								
Engineer's signature								

Defects schedule				
Date	Observations	Noted	Diagnosed cause of defect	Initials

Establishment .... Logbook

Site .... Page No 8

Installation .... Serial No 1

Frequency months

Maintenance sheet for condenser water
circulation system monthly tasks

When maintenance task is satisfactorily completed the operative is to tick the box opposite. If task cannot be completed due to mechanical failure, insert a cross in the box opposite and note defect on the observation sheet.

Job Description	Date of inspection							
1. Condenser water circulation Pump No. 1								
a) isolate electrical supplies locally.								
b) remove guards, inspect for rust and make good as necessary.								
c) wipe clean motor, shaft, pump casing and parts as appropriate.								
d) check all bearings and adjust as necessary.								
e) lubricate pump bearings with.............								
f) shots of grease type								
g) check belt drives for correct alignment and tension and adjust as required.								
h) check pump glands for excessive leakage, adjust or replace as required.								
i) clean drip cups and rod through as required.								
j) check tightness of all holding down bolts and anti-vibration mountings. Realign if required.								
k) bring pump back into service.								
2. Condenser water circulation Pump No. 2								
Where dual pump installations exist draw up additional maintenance sheet and implement maintenance function.								
Engineer's signature								

Job description	Date of inspection							
3. Dosing pump for chemical A **a) check pump bearing and where not sealed for life oil or grease to manufacturers instructions.** **b) disconnect pump discharge and run for set time discharging contents into measuring container to check duty remains satisfactory.** **c) tighten pump holding down assembly on top of chemical treatment tank.** **4. Dosing pump for chemical B** **Where more than one dosing set is installed draw up maintenance sheets for each system and implement maintenance function.** **5. Strainer** **a) remove strainer basket, insert standby basket, bring service back on line, empty and clean basket.** **6. Pressure gauges and thermometers** **a) clean all glass dial gauges and mercury in glass stem thermometers to ensure clarity of reading.**								
Engineer's signature								

Defects schedule				
Date	Observations	Noted	Diagnosed cause of defect	Initials

Defects schedule				
Date	Observations	Noted	Diagnosed cause of defect	Initials

Establishment .... Logbook

Site .... Page No 8

Installation .... Serial No 2

Frequency 6 monthly

Maintenance sheet for condenser water
circulation system - 6 monthly tasks

When maintenance task is satisfactorily completed the operative is to tick the box opposite. If task cannot be completed due to mechanical failure, insert a cross in the box opposite and note defect on the observation sheet.

Job Description	Date of inspection							
1. Valves a) clean all valve spindles of dust or deposits. b) operate valve through two full cycles from fully open to fully closed and reset to precise original position. c) inspect gland and adjust gland nut as required. Repack gland if required. d) lubricate valve is required by manufacturer.								
2. 3-Way control valve a) check valve spindle for signs of wear and distortion. Replace as necessary. b) check glands and adjust as necessary. c) check table terminals and tighten or check pneumatic tubing and tighten nipples if necessary.								
3. Automatic air vents a) isolate feed to AAV, dismantle, remove float and clean float and needles. Clean ports and needle seats. b) blow through discharge lines.								
Engineer's signature								

Job description	Date of inspection							
4. Drains and sample points a) open all drain lines and sample points to blow clear. Check discharges to ensure lines freely drain over gully to waste.								
5. a) remove flow monitor, inspect and operate paddle. Chemically clean and replace. b) check and tighten cable terminals.								
6. Flow monitor a) gain access to NRV clack and inspect for freedom of operation scoring or erosion. Renew disc if required and reassemble.								
7. Conductivity cell a) remove conductivity cell from pipeline, inspect and clean as recommended by manufacturer.								
8. Thermometers a) check all thermometers pockets for thermoconductive paste and replenish as required.								
Engineer's signature								

Defects schedule				
Date	Observations	Noted	Diagnosed cause of defect	Initials

Defects schedule				
Date	Observations	Noted	Diagnosed cause of defect	Initials

Establishment . . . . Logbook

Site . . . . Page No 8

Installation . . . . Serial No 3

Maintenance sheet for condenser water
circulation system yearly or as necessary

Frequency yearly
or as necessary

When maintenance task is satisfactorily completed the operative is to tick the box opposite. If task cannot be completed due to mechanical failure, insert a cross in the box opposite and note defect on the observation sheet.

Job description	Date of inspection							
1. Internal pipe inspections a) when system is drained for seasonal cleaning, remove inspection flanges and note condition of pipe interior.								
2. Pressure gauges a) remove pressure gauges and recalibrate or exchange for a recalibrated gauge.								
3. Condenser a) remove end plates. Clean off any signs of corrosion from tube plates and treat as recommended by manufacturer. b) rod through all tubes with the rodding brush and apply hose to clean out debris. c) reassemble and put into service.								
4. Thermometer pockets a) remove all thermometer pockets and inspect for fouling. If required chemically clean pocket. b) replace pocket, repack with thermoconductive paste and insert thermometer.								
Engineer's signature								

Defects schedule				
Date	Observations	Noted	Diagnosed cause of defect	Initials

Appendix 5 – Empty times for cooling tower ponds (approx)

Pond	Capacity	Cooling tower drain valves sizes mm (inch)							
		25 (1.0)		38 (1.5)		50 (2.0)		63 (2.5)	
		Tank depths		Tank depths		Tank depths		Tank depths	
litres	(gals)	0.5 m	1.0 m	0.5 m	1.0 m	0.5 m	1.0 m	0.5 m	1.0 m
150	(35)	5 min	-	-	-	-	-	-	-
259	(57)	8 min	5 min	5 min	-	-	-	-	-
345	(76)	11 min	8 min	7 min	-	-	-	-	-
968	(213)	30 min	20 min	15 min	10 min	10 min	5 min	5 min	-
1,500	(330)	50 min	35 min	20 min	15 min	15 min	10 min	10 min	5 min
2,800	(616)	1 hr 30 min	1 hr 00 min	40 min	30 min	25 min	15 min	15 min	10 min
5,500	(1,210)	3 hr 00 min	2 hr 00 min	1 hr 15 min	1 hr 00 min	45 min	30 min	30 min	20 min
8,500	(1,870)	4 hr 30 min	3 hr 00 min	2 hr 00 min	1 hr 30 min	1 hr 15 min	45 min	45 min	30 min
11,000	(2,420)	6 hr 00 min	4 hr 00 min	2 hr 30 min	2 hr 00 min	1 hr 30 min	1 hr 00 min	1 hr 00 min	40 min

Times assume no hose and gate valve.

Notes

1. Ball type valves should be specified to minimise "clogging".
2. The drain from the gully must be of sufficient size to take the flow from the pond.

Appendix 6 – Cooling towers – operational checks

6.1 These tasks should be carried out weekly. Usually, visual inspection is sufficient.

Evaporative cooling system operational checks

6.2 The specimen logbook, page 2, details the checks and tasks to be covered. It is expected that the engineer will exercise discretion (as to the degree of involvement) where weekly checks are indicated. The tasks listed entail observation from close inspection and do not require dismantling or draining of plant, etc. (More detailed examination is covered under routine maintenance.) For instance, a "pond inspection" on a weekly basis is intended to be a visual inspection of the pond to establish the following:

a) correct operating water level;

b) water appears clean and free from slime, with no foreign matter floating or submerged.

Make-up water operational checks

6.3 Readings and tests as shown in the logbook page 3 should be carried out on a weekly basis. The readings are required to ensure that the minimum amount of water is used, and that water treatment is maintained to reduce the risk of microbial growth and to suit the chemical treatment programme.

System water quality operational tests

6.4 The tests given in the logbook page 5 should be carried out weekly to ensure proper control of the water treatment programme so as to restrict the development of *Legionella pneumophila*, the accumulation of scale, slime, sludge, etc.

Equipment checks

6.5 Each item of equipment should be checked using the senses of sight, touch, smell and hearing as applicable. This type of check will complement the readings taken from instruments and will allow comprehensive details to be recorded on the log sheet. Where such checks show that corrective measures can be carried out quickly and efficiently at the time of the inspection (using minimal tools and equipment), this should be done. Where the checks identify more time-consuming remedial action, with the use of specific plant and materials, the work should be carried out at the earliest opportunity following inspection. A preventive planned maintenance scheme should avoid the need for unforeseen, substantial maintenance tasks being identified during the weekly inspections.

6.6 Typical observations and checks are listed below:

a. pond:

  (i) check water level is properly marked on the pond and is maintained;

  (ii) check overflow is clear;

  (iii) check ball valve flow and proper shut-off;

  (iv) check water for leaves and foreign matter;

  (v) check for slime and signs of scaling;

  (vi) check for leaks;

  (vii) check for signs of corrosion, for example rusting, algae blistering, oxidisation, etc;

  (viii) check clear visibility of sump;

  (ix) check screen in pond and clean as necessary;

  (x) check drains are free;

  (xi) check discharge from pack for uniformity;

b. tower casing:

  (i) check for rattles and vibration;

  (ii) check the casing for water and air leaks while in operation;

  (iii) check for drift from tower discharge;

  (iv) check for signs of corrosion, for example rusting, blistering, oxidisation, etc;

  (v) check paint or protective coating for damage;

  (vi) check louvres and screens for leaves, growth and other deterioration;

c. tower internals:

  (i) check pack for correct location, alignment, seal and absence of distortion;

  (ii) check pack for condition and signs of deterioration, scale, algae, slime, poor water flow/coverage;

  (iii) check casing and inside structure for signs of corrosion, rusting, blistering and oxidisation;

  (iv) check sprays, sparge or troughs for efficient operation and uniformity of distribution of water over pack when operating;

  (v) check drift eliminator for correct location, alignment and lack of distortion and seal;

  (vi) check drift eliminator for signs of deterioration, scale, algae, slime or blockage;

d. cooling tower fan:

  (i) check for noise vibration and free running;

  (ii) check drive method where applicable for correct adjustment, alignment and operation;

  (iii) check cage, guard and screen for corrosion and proper location and fixing;

  (iv) check motor full-load current and record;

  (v) check condition of impeller, shaft, housing, scroll, shaft, bearing and supports, etc;

e. sump immersion heater and trace heating:

  (i) check power available and isolator position;

  (ii) check operation manually;

  (iii) check thermostat setting;

f. pipework distribution system:

  (i) check for signs of leaks;

  (ii) check for signs of corrosion;

  (iii) check for vibration;

  (iv) vent all air cocks and check all AAVs and discharge lines;

  (v) check all drains are operable and gulleys are clear;

g. manual valves and cocks:

  (i) check all valve glands for leaks or solid deposits collecting around spindle;

  (ii) check for the correct setting of all valves (fully open, closed, partially open, etc);

h. automatic 3-way control valves and associated equipment:

  (i) check 3-way control valve fully operational;

  (ii) check 3-way valve maintenance bypass valve is closed save for bleed facility;

  (iii) check for positive shut-off as applicable;

  (iv) re-establish automatic control, calibrate detector and set to design temperature;

j. strainer:

  (i) compare system flow to bypass flow and assess if strainer might be partially blocked;

  (ii) check that spare strainer basket is available;

k. circulating pump:

  (i) check each pump for smooth running and freedom from noise and vibration;

  (ii) check bearings for grease and high temperature;

  (iii) check shaft and drives for signs of wear;

  (iv) check belts and pulley for correct alignment and tension of belts;

  (v) check guards for proper fixing and absence of vibration and corrosion;

  (vi) check clearance of guards for free operation;

  (vii) check glands for excessive leakage and check drip lines are clear and free draining to gulley;

  (viii) operate stop locks and auto-change facility as applicable;

  (ix) operate each pump via on/off/auto switch to prove operation;

  (x) measure suction and discharge pressures, record and compare with design. Increase in pressure difference will indicate reduction in flow, possibly caused by strainers or condenser tube fouling. Note observations;

  (xi) record hours run for each pump;

  (xii) check pump mounting condition and effectiveness;

  (xiii) check foundations, securing bolts and pump alignment with pipework and assess any movement or creeping;

m. condenser:

  (i) vent condenser via air cocks to relieve any air pockets;

  (ii) measure condenser water inlet and outlet pressures and record;

  (iii) record condenser pressure differential and compare with design and flow as measured in (h) above and assess any fouling;

         (iv) record water entry and leaving temperatures;

         (v) record refrigeration machine full-load current associated with water temperature difference and compare with manufacturer's chart to assess load-cross check with flow and temperature difference readings taken;

n. flow monitor:

         (i) stop/start pumps and check free operation and ready switching of flow monitor;

         (ii) check refrigeration machine shuts down on no-flow;

         (iii) check action of "delay-on" timer to refrigeration circuit and others as applicable;

p. dosing system(s) – for each system:

Checking frequency will depend on dosing rates and capacity of the chemical containers/drums, for example, small containers may be exhausted in as little as three days

         (i) check contents of drum(s) and note volume remaining;

         (ii) top up drum(s) with water treatment chemicals and record new volume of contents;

         (iii) manually operate dosing pump(s) and check for correct operation and freedom from vibration, etc;

         (iv) manually override controller(s) to cycle pump(s) automatically, check controller calibration, reset and leave under automatic control;

Initially while the plant is settling down, thereafter less frequently

         (v) check dosing pump(s) duty/calibration manually;

         (vi) check setting and operation of any timers.

Other publications in this series

(Given below are details of all Health Technical Memoranda available from HMSO. HTMs marked (*) are currently being revised, those marked (†) are out of print. Some HTMs in preparation at the time of publication of this HTM are also listed.)

1	Anti-static precautions: rubber, plastics and fabrics*†
2	Anti-static precautions: flooring in anaesthetising areas (and data processing rooms)*, 1977.
3	–
4	–
5	Steam boiler plant instrumentation†
6	Protection of condensate systems: filming amines†
2007	Electrical services: supply and distribution, 1993.
8	–
9	–
10	Sterilizers*†
2011	Emergency electrical services, 1992.
12	–
13	–
2014	Abatement of electrical interference, 1993.
15	Patient/nurse call systems†
16	–
17	Health building engineering installations: commissioning and associated activities, 1978.
18	Facsimile telegraphy: possible applications in DGHs†
19	Facsimile telegraphy: the transmission of pathology reports within a hospital – a case study†
2020	Electrical safety code for low voltage systems, 1993.
2021	Electrical safety code for high voltage systems, 1993.
22	Piped medical gases, medical compressed air and medical vacuum installations*†
22 Supp.	Permit to work system: for piped medical gases etc†
23	Access and accommodation for engineering services†
24	–
25	–
26	Commissioning of oil, gas and dual fired boilers: with notes on design, operation and maintenance†
27	Cold water supply storage and mains distribution* [Revised version will deal with water storage and distribution], 1978.
28 to 39	–
41 to 53	–

Component Data Base (HTMs 54 to 70)

54.1	User manual, 1993.
55	Windows, 1989.
56	Partitions, 1989.
57	Internal glazing, 1989.
58	Internal doorsets, 1989.
59	Ironmongery, 1989.
60	Ceilings, 1989.
61	Flooring, 1989.
62	Demountable storage systems, 1989.
63	Fitted storage systems, 1989.
64	Sanitary assemblies, 1989.
65	Signs†
66	Cubicle curtain track, 1989.
67	Laboratory fitting-out system, 1993.
68	Ducts and panel assemblies, 1993.
69	Protection, 1993.
70	Fixings, 1993.
71 to 80	–

Firecode

81	Firecode: fire precautions in new hospitals, 1987.
81	Supp 1, 1993.
82	Firecode: alarm and detection systems, 1989.
83	Fire safety in health care premises: general fire precautions*†
85	[Revision to Home Office draft guidance in preparation]
86	Firecode: assessing fire risks in existing hospital wards, 1987.
87	Firecode: textiles and furniture, 1993.
88	Fire safety in health care premises: guide to fire precautions in NHS housing in the community for mentally handicapped/ill people, 1986.

New HTMs in preparation

Lifts
Combined heat and power
Telecommunications (telephone exchanges)
Washers for sterile production
Ventilation in healthcare premises
Risk management and quality assurance

Health Technical Memoranda published by HMSO can be purchased from HMSO Bookshops in London (post orders to PO Box 276, SW8 5DT), Edinburgh, Belfast, Manchester, Birmingham and Bristol, or through good booksellers. HMSO provide a copy service for publications which are out of print; and a standing order service.

Enquiries about Health Technical Memoranda (but not orders) should be addressed to: NHS Estates, Department of Health, Marketing and Publications Unit, 1 Trevelyan Square, Boar Lane, Leeds LS1 6AE.

About NHS Estates

NHS Estates is an Executive Agency of the Department of Health and is involved with all aspects of health estate management, development and maintenance. The Agency has a dynamic fund of knowledge which it has acquired during 30 years of working in the field. Using this knowledge NHS Estates has developed products which are unique in range and depth. These are described below.

NHS Estates also makes its experience available to the field through its consultancy services.

Enquiries should be addressed to: NHS Estates, Department of Health, 1 Trevelyan Square, Boar Lane, Leeds LS1 6AE. Tel: 0532 547000.

Some other NHS Estates products

Activity DataBase – a computerised system for defining the activities which have to be accommodated in spaces within health buildings. *NHS Estates*

Design Guides – complementary to Health Building Notes, Design Guides provide advice for planners and designers about subjects not appropriate to the Health Building Notes series. *HMSO*

Estatecode – user manual for managing a health estate. Includes a recommended methodology for property appraisal and provides a basis for integration of the estate into corporate business planning. *HMSO*

Capricode – a framework for the efficient management of capital projects from inception to completion. *HMSO*

Concode – outlines proven methods of selecting contracts and commissioning consultants. Both parts reflect official policy on contract procedures. *HMSO*

Works Information Management System – a computerised information system for estate management tasks, enabling tangible assets to be put into the context of servicing requirements. *NHS Estates*

Option Appraisal Guide – advice during the early stages of evaluating a proposed capital building scheme. Supplementary guidance to Capricode. *HMSO*

Health Building Notes – advice for project teams procuring new buildings and adapting or extending existing buildings. *HMSO*

Health Facilities Notes – debate current and topical issues of concern across all areas of healthcare provision. *HMSO*

Health Guidance Notes – an occasional series of publications which respond to changes in Department of Health policy or reflect changing NHS operational management. Each deals with a specific topic and is complementary to a related Health Technical Memorandum. *HMSO*

Encode – shows how to plan and implement a policy of energy efficiency in a building. *HMSO*

Firecode – for policy, technical guidance and specialist aspects of fire precautions. *HMSO*

Nucleus – standardised briefing and planning system combining appropriate standards of clinical care and service with maximum economy in capital and running costs. *NHS Estates*

Concise – Software support for managing the capital programme. Compatible with Capricode. *NHS Estates*

Items noted "HMSO" can be purchased from HMSO Bookshops in London (post orders to PO Box 276, SW8 5DT), Edinburgh, Belfast, Manchester, Birmingham and Bristol or through good booksellers. Details of their standing order service are given at the front of this publication.

Enquiries about NHS Estates products should be addressed to: NHS Estates, Marketing and Publications Unit, Department of Health, 1 Trevelyan Square, Boar Lane, Leeds LS1 6AE.

NHS Estates consultancy service

Designed to meet a range of needs from advice on the oversight of estates management functions to a much fuller collaboration for particularly innovative or exemplary projects.

Enquiries should be addressed to: NHS Estates Consultancy Service (address as above).

Printed in the United Kingdom for HMSO.
Dd. 297566, C15, 12/93, 3396/4, 5673, 264467.